T0358848

Nursing Skills in Safety and Protection

People should be cared for in a safe environment that is protected from internal and external harm. This quick reference guide covers vital practical skills for nurses including:

- Emergency management and resuscitation
- The safe and accurate administration of medicines
- Infection control
- The anatomy and physiology of skin and temperature regulation
- Personal care
- Wound care.

This competency-based text covers relevant key concepts, anatomy and physiology, lifespan matters, assessment and nursing skills. To support your learning, it also includes learning outcomes, concept map summaries, activities, questions and scenarios with sample answers, and critical reflection thinking points.

Quick and easy to reference, this short, clinically focused guide is ideal for use on placements or for revision. It is suitable for pre-registration nurses, students on the nursing associate programme and newly qualified nurses.

Sheila Cunningham is an Associate Professor in Adult Nursing at Middlesex University, UK. She has a breadth of experience teaching nurses both pre- and post-registration and she supports mentors supporting students in practice. She is also a Middlesex University Teaching Fellow and holds a Principal Fellowship at the Higher Education Academy. She is currently programme leader for the BSc European nursing.

Tina Moore is a Senior Lecturer in Adult Nursing at Middlesex University, UK. She teaches nursing assessment, clinical skills and acute care interventions for both pre-qualifying and post-qualifying nurses. Her interests are in simulated learning approaches and Objective Structured Clinical examination (OSCE) as a teaching and assessment method. She has authored a number of books and articles. She is also a Middlesex University Teaching Fellow.

Skills in Nursing Practice

Series editors
Tina Moore, *Middlesex University, UK*
Sheila Cunningham, *Middlesex University, UK*

This series of competency-based pocket guides covers relevant key concepts, anatomy and physiology, lifespan matters, assessment and nursing skills for good clinical practice in a range of areas from safety and protection to promoting homeostasis. To support your learning, they include learning outcomes, concept map summaries, activities, questions and scenarios with sample answers, and critical reflection thinking points.

Quick and easy to reference, these short, skills-focused texts are ideal for use on placements or for revision. They are ideal for pre-registration nurses, students on the nursing associate programme and newly qualified nurses feeling in need of a little revision.

List of titles

Nursing Skills in Professional and Practice Contexts
Tina Moore and Sheila Cunningham

Nursing Skills in Safety and Protection
Sheila Cunningham and Tina Moore

Nursing Skills in Nutrition, Hydration and Elimination
Sheila Cunningham and Tina Moore

For more information about this series, please visit: www.routledge.com/Skills-in-Nursing-Practice/book-series/SNP

Nursing Skills in Safety and Protection

Sheila Cunningham and Tina Moore

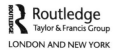

Routledge
Taylor & Francis Group

LONDON AND NEW YORK

First published 2020
by Routledge
2 Park Square, Milton Park, Abingdon, Oxon OX14 4RN

and by Routledge
52 Vanderbilt Avenue, New York, NY 10017

Routledge is an imprint of the Taylor & Francis Group, an informa business

British Library Cataloguing-in-Publication Data
A catalogue record for this book is available from the
British Library

Library of Congress Cataloging-in-Publication Data
A catalog record has been requested for this book

ISBN: 978-1-138-47940-1 (hbk)
ISBN: 978-1-138-47941-8 (pbk)
ISBN: 978-1-351-06578-8 (ebk)

Typeset in Stone Serif
by Wearset Ltd, Boldon, Tyne and Wear

Contents

Figures

Introduction to the Skills in Nursing Practice series

This particular book is one in a series of six *'Nursing Skills in ...'*.

Book 1 *Professional and Practice Context*
Book 2 *Protection and Safety*
Book 3 *Nutrition, Hydration and Elimination*
Book 4 *Control and Coordination*
Book 5 *Cardiorespiratory Assessment and Monitoring*
Book 6 *Mobility and Support*

These books are designed to be used in clinical practice and can be used not only for reference but also as an invaluable revision tool. There is a continuing emphasis on skills acquisition and development particularly within nursing. This is accompanied by the increasing understanding of the necessity to effectively and efficiently integrate theory and clinical skill competence-based learning. In doing so, this ensures that nurses have the best opportunity to become 'fit to practise' and develop key employability skills. Therefore, each chapter has been linked to the *Future Nurse Proficiencies* (Nursing and Midwifery Council 2018a), which will enable you, as the nurse, to map your skills development in relation to the standards set by the professional body.

The structure of each chapter within the books draws on constructivist pedagogical approaches and assimilation theory. Each chapter has interlinking ideas and information through the use of concept maps. It is anticipated that the use of key words and connections will deepen and enhance these linkages from the concepts, drawing on general and specific aspects of a topic, and therefore promote active learning.

Concept maps are pictures or graphic representations that will help you to organise and represent knowledge of a subject.

1

This is achieved through helping you to link, differentiate and relate concepts to each other. They (concept maps) begin with a main idea (or concept) and then branch out to show how that main idea can be broken down into specific topics. They can also visually represent relationships between concepts and ideas in a quick, easy-to-understand format. Concept mapping is becoming increasingly popular as a means of teaching and learning within education. The introduction of concept maps will provide a quick summary **with** additional key information of the material read in the *Clinical Skills for Nursing Practice* book. We have also included related anatomy and physiology together with lifespan matters.

The end of each chapter has questions (answers also provided) in the format of a quiz. This will help you to test your knowledge, understanding and application of the content. There is also the opportunity for you to critically reflect on your learning using a SMART (specific, measureable, achievable, realistic and time-frame) format. From this you should then be able to clearly identify areas for future development and learning.

These pocket-size books are designed not only to help develop further your clinical skills (practice and knowledge), but also to improve your key transferrable skills, enabling them to advance your employability skills, i.e. problem solving, analytical and critical thinking, and team working. Therefore another aim for each book is to concentrate on scaffolding learning, as a result supporting, promoting and developing autonomous learning, questioning (informed) and critical thinking. The use of concept mapping allows reorganisation of information in a visual manner to promote critical thinking in the student nurse. Through concept mapping students can see how ideas/patient care needs and the interrelationships that exist promote critical thinking in relation to clinical practice.

The books within this series are not designed to be comprehensive textbooks. It is the practice companion of the *Clinical Skills for Nursing Practice*, and is designed to be used together with that book. The design of these 'pocket-size' books will enable students/readers to use them as a resource while working within and outside of clinical practice.

Tina Moore and Sheila Cunningham

Introduction and overview

Protecting patients and ensuring safety are key to quality nursing care. This is more than adhering to legal responsibilities (such as the Health and Safety at Work Act 1973), but extends to core nursing activities and especially patient-focused care. Protection and safety are wide reaching, extending from managing emergency situations, prescribing medicines and medicines management, to infection control, and addressing skin care and integrity. The Nursing and Midwifery Council (NMC 2018b) assert that nurses have a responsibility for safety and protecting patients and the public, but also themselves. The Code (of professional practice) summarises this with the framework for practice intended to signify what good nursing and midwifery practice looks like. It puts the interests of patients and service users first, is safe and effective, and promotes trust through professionalism. There are several areas of nursing practice that support protection and safety, and ultimately everything nurses do for patients is about safe practice, but protection, however, this short book has four areas: emergency procedures and lifesaving events, medicines management, infection control and skin integrity. It ought be read in conjunction with the other books in the series, which divide up knowledge and skills into chapters intended to build up your knowledge and key information to practise holistic care safely.

CHAPTER 1

Emergency care and management

Tina Moore

Overview

Emergency care and management entail early recognition of clinical deterioration through the use of the ABCDE assessment model and effective management of a patient suffering from the most common life-threatening clinical conditions (e.g. shock, burns, anaphylaxis). It also includes life support through airway management, basic life support and advanced life support.

Link to *Future Nurse Proficiencies* (Nursing and Midwifery Council [NMC] 2018a)

Platform 4 Providing and evaluating care: specifically 4.13
This demonstrates the knowledge, skills and confidence to provide first aid procedures and basic life support.
Skills annexe B, 10.5: use evidence-based, best practice approaches for meeting needs for care and support at the end of life, accurately assessing the person's capacity for independence and self-care and initiating appropriate interventions.

Expected knowledge

- Anatomy and physiology of the respiratory, circulatory, renal and neurological systems
- Methods of assessment
- Fundamentals of basic and advanced life support
- Key general ethical and legal principles

Introduction

In the UK, similar to other countries, there has been increasing emphasis on safety issues. The internet has become a welcome source of accessing immediate information. There is a wealth of evidence-based material (some formulated as clinical guidelines) available. Useful information can be found from sources such as:

- National Institute for Health and Care Excellence (NICE)
- National Patient Safety Agency (NSPA)
- Department of Health (DH)
- Resuscitation guidelines
- British Thoracic Society Publications
- Scottish Intercollegiate Guidelines Network (SIGN)

The healthcare needs of patients within the hospital setting and the community are becoming increasingly complex. This is for a variety of reasons: people are living longer so more have experienced the effects of the ageing process; modern technology; and medications prolonging life. This requires healthcare professionals, including nurses, to have the appropriate knowledge and skill to preserve life, relieve suffering, limit disability and promote recovery.

Content

ABCDE assessment	Recognition of the deteriorating patient	Airway management
Basic life support	Early defibrillation	Emergency first aid
Advanced life support (ALS) and professional issues (adult)	ALS and professional issues (paediatric)	Post-resuscitation care

Learning outcomes

- Demonstrate knowledge and understanding of the use of a systematic approach (ABCDE) in the assessment of an acutely or critically ill patient, or a patient who is clinically deteriorating

- Recognise the signs that indicate a patient is deteriorating
- Discuss the procedure for basic and advanced life support (adult and paediatric)
- Identify key professional issues in relation to resuscitation
- Provide emergency first aid for a variety of situations (including bleeding, burns, anaphylaxis, shock and choking)

Key background

Unlike most other healthcare professionals, nurses are in more contact with patients, and are best placed to identify problems and initiate actions early. Early recognition of patient deterioration can be determined only through effective observations and a structured and systematic approach to that assessment. This should enable a more accurate appraisal of the patient's clinical condition, and the initiation of appropriate and prompt and appropriate management. (particularly the use of defibrillation) has been linked to positive patient outcomes.

ABCDE ASSESSMENT

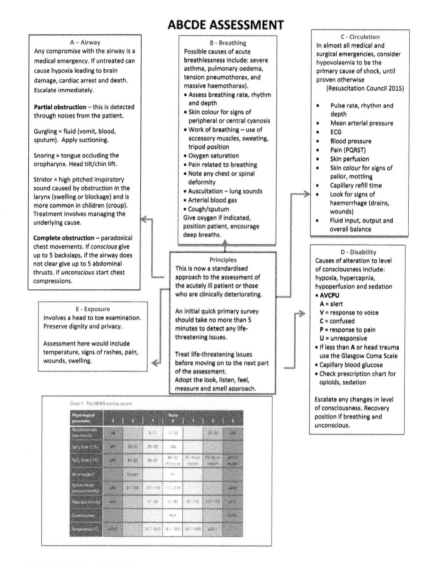

FIGURE 1.1 ABCDE assessment

EARLY RECOGNITION OF THE DETERIORATING PATIENT

Primary survey – quick initial 5-minute scan to determine immediate threats to life.

Secondary survey – once stable, more in-depth assessment/investigations.

- Signs and symptoms
- Allergies
- Medications
- Pertinent medical history
- Last oral intake
- Events leading to illness

CORE PHYSICAL ASSESSMENT SKILLS

Inspection (vision, hearing, smell)

Palpation (touch)

Percussion (sound through tapping)

Auscultation (listening through a stethoscope – lung, heart bowel sounds)

PRIMARY SURVEY (LOOK/LISTEN/FEEL/ SMELL/MEASURE)

A Airway (patency/partial or full obstruction)

B Breathing (respiratory status)

C Circulation (Ccirculatory/cardiac status)

D Disability (level of consciousness/pain assessment

E Exposure (head to toe physical assessment)

SIGNS OF DETERIORATON

EARLY   LATE

EARLY	LATE
Tachypnoea	Bradypnoea
Retraction (in children)	Bradycardia
Tachycardia	Hypotension
Pallor	Mottled/poor
Irritability	perfusion
	Confusion

Physiological measures

- Respiratory rate
- Oxygen saturation
- Systolic blood pressure
- Heart rate
- Level of consciousness
- Temperature

MAJOR COMPONENTS OF A COMPREHENSIVE ASSESSMENT

- Systematic approach
- Evidence-based approach
- Age considerations
- Knowledge of normal parameters (with consideration to chronic pathophysiological changes)
- Baseline of level of patient wellness
- Knowledge of physiology
- Knowledge of pathophysiology
- Past and current medical history
- Patient appearance at time of assessment

Do not use the National Early Warning Score (**NEWS**) for the pregnant woman as this has limitations. Use Modified Early Obstetric Warning Score (**MEOWS**) and for children, the Paediatric Early Warning Score (**PEWS**).

| Vital signs monitoring and trend analysis | ⇒ | Early detection (respiratory rate/heart rate) | ⇒ | Early intervention | ⇒ | Improving patient safety |

FIGURE 1.2 Early recognition of the deteriorating patient

EMERGENCY FIRST AID

BLEEDING

- Arterial (bright red and spurting)
- Venous (dark red and oozing)
- Capillary (trickling)

Immediate intervention

S Sit or lay down
E Examine the injury
E Elevate the wound (if a limb then above heart level)
P Pressure (*direct* – 10 minutes continuous / *Indirect* – compress brachial or femoral artery with a pad/clean cloth)

If blood soaks through the material, don't remove it, instead add more on top and continue the pressure.
Raise the limb.
DO NOT apply a tourniquet.
Use disposable gloves.
If anything is embedded in the wound, leave it and do not apply pressure on it.

ANAPHYLAXIS

This is a severe life-threatening, generalised or systemic hypersensitive reaction (e.g. food, drugs, insect venom) causing an overwhelming inflammatory response.

Symptoms include: swelling of upper airways, stridor, cyanosis, hypotension, confusion, rash.

- Fowler's position (unless hypotensive)
- (P) airway management
- High flow oxygen
- Obtain information regarding allergies/past medical history
- Adrenaline (some may carry epipen) intramuscular – this can be repeated after 5 minutes if no improvement

BURNS

- **Dry heat** (direct contact e.g. flame). Stop the burning process as soon as possible.
  Do not remove anything stuck into the burnt skin.
  Use lukewarm running water for 20 minutes to cool the burn.
  Remove appropriate clothing/jewellery.
  Cover burn with clingfilm/non-adhesive dressing.
- **Wet heat** (boiling water and other very hot liquids)
  First aid as dry heat.
- **Chemical** (e.g. sulphuric acid)
  Remove any contaminated clothing unless stuck on skin.
  Brush off dry chemical from skin.
  Use lukewarm water to remove chemical from skin for at least 20 minutes.
- **Radiation** (e.g. sunburn/tanning beds)
  Remove source of burn.
  Cool burn with lukewarm water.
  Give water to drink if conscious.
- **Electrical**
  Switch off power supply if in contact.
  If required, use dry insulating material e.g. wood to make the scene safe (remove electrical source).
  Try to cool exit and entry wounds with water.
  As per dry heat.
  Patient MUST be assessed by a doctor.

1st degree – burnt epidermis
Redness/swelling and pain

2nd degree – burnt epidermis and dermis
Blisters/swelling and severe pain

3rd degree – all layers of skin, and fat, muscle and bone affected
Dry white/black areas and no pain

First degree burn

Second degree burn

Third degree burn

CHOKING

Symptoms	Procedure
Unable to speak/cough	1. Encourage cough.
Grasping throat	2. If they cannot cough, shout for help.
Pale and cyanotic	3. Give five back blows (help patient to bend forward). With palm of hand, hit patient firmly between the shoulder blades. Check to see if the obstruction has come out.
Distressed	
Unconscious	4. If nothing comes out, repeat up to five times.
	5. Five abdominal thrusts (if airway completely obstructed and patient cannot cough). Stand behind patient. Link your hands at their upper abdomen with your lower hand clenched in a fist. Push firmly inwards and upwards.
	6. Check obstruction.
	7. Repeat up to five times.
	8. Call for ambulance (if in community) and repeat steps 2–7.
	9. Check level of consciousness throughout. If they are not breathing, start CPR.

SHOCK

This is potentially a life-threatening condition caused by a lack of oxygen supply to the body tissues.

Cardiogenic (acute coronary syndrome, heart failure)
Hypovolaemic (loss of body fluids, e.g. bleeding, dehydration, vomiting)
Septic (severe infection)
Anaphylactic (severe allergic reaction)
Neurogenic (head/spinal injury)

Stages:
1. **Compensatory** (increased heart rate, slightly decreased or normal blood pressure, pale/clammy skin)
2. **Progressive** (tachycardia, hypotension, tachypnoea, cyanosis, clammy skin, dizziness)
3. **Refactory** (slow, laboured breathing, unconsciousness, multi-organ failure)

Lay patient flat with legs elevated
Keep patient warm
Monitor ABCDE
Treatment will be dependent upon the cause

FIGURE 1.3 Emergency first aid

EARLY
DEFIBRILLATION

> - AED are located in many public places.
> - Makes it possible to defibrillate much earlier than professional help arrives.
> - AED can also detect arrhythmias that have potential to be reverted.
> - Important to follow the voice prompts.

Automated External Defibrillator

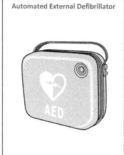

Shockable rhythms

Ventricular tachycardia
Rapid ventricular activity. Impulse outside of normal conducting pathway. Due to rate, cardiac output is reduced.

Ventricular fibrillation
Chaotic. Rhythm cannot be determined. No synchronisation of blood pumped out of ventricles.

Safety issues

Children under 1 year – DO NOT USE

Children older than 8 years – can be used as per adult

Fluids – ensure patient or those delivering the shock are not next to loose fluids

Supplemental oxygen – remove from the patient at least one metre before delivering the shock

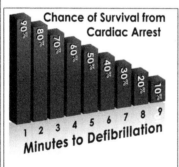

Chance of Survival from Cardiac Arrest

90% 80% 70% 60% 50% 40% 30% 20% 10%

1 2 3 4 5 6 7 8 9
Minutes to Defibrillation

Procedure

1. Open the case and remove AED
2. Switch AED on
3. If more than one person, continue with CPR – minimise disruption to chest compression
4. Other person should follow the voice/visual prompts step by step
5. Use defibrillation pads to **dry** skin on patient's chest (excessive hair should be shaved) – 2× for adult, 1 on sternum and 1 between shoulder blades for child
6. Analysis of heart rhythm – NO-ONE to touch patient or bed
7. 'No shock advised' – continue CRP
8. 'Shock advised' – put finger over shock button
9. 'Deliver shock now' – say 'stand clear shock to be given', then press the shock button
10. When sure everyone is clear state – 'delivering shock now'
11. Resume CPR as per guidelines
12. If patient shows signs of life – AED with notify
13. If no signs of life, AED with restart the process every 2 minutes

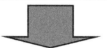

Additional concerns

Remove bra or cut through middle to expose centre of chest.

Remove or cut any jewellery. Cover body piercings (do not put pad over).

Ensure at least one pad distance between the two pads.

FIGURE 1.4 Basic life support

AIRWAY MANAGEMENT

The brain needs a constant supply of oxygen for survival. A non-patent airway is a life-threating EMERGENCY situation

Causes of obstruction
- Foreign body
- Depressed consciousness, e.g. head injury, opiates, alcohol causing displacement of tongue, soft palate, epiglottis
- Fluid (blood/vomit)
- Swelling/oedema of the face, throat, tongue (allergic reaction)
- Swelling/inflammatory processes (burns/smoke)
- Displacement of artificial airway adjuncts
- Facial trauma

Airway management
The 'sniffing position' (optimum position to open airway) – head extension and flexion of neck on body

Head tilt and chin lift
Hyperextend neck (adult) – not for suspected cervical spinal injury use **jaw thrust** (adult/child) instead

Head neutral alignment (infant)

Don't hyperextend neck and do not push on soft tissues under chin (child)

Suctioning
If the above does not work – use **airway adjuncts** (below)

Give **high concentration of oxygen** (maintain oxygen saturations above 90%)
Tracheal intubation may be required

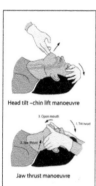

Head tilt –chin lift manoeuvre

Jaw thrust manoeuvre

Signs of airway obstruction

Patency occurs when the patient is speaking clearly without distress.

Signs would include partial tracheal tug, irritability and agitation, reduced level of consciousness. DO NOT rely on cyanosis or reduced oxygen saturation levels as these are VERY late signs.

Partial obstruction (noises)

➢ Snoring (pharynx is partially obstructed by soft palate or tongue). Put in 'sniffing' position. If unconscious, place in left lateral position.

➢ Gurgling (fluid in the upper airway e.g. vomitus, sputum). Suction patient.

➢ Stridor (a harsh high pitch noise, commonly occurring on inspiration)

Complete obstruction

➢ No breath sounds.

➢ Paradoxical chest and abdominal movements ('see-saw' respiration).

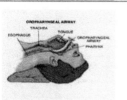

Nasopharyngeal airway (semi- or unconscious). Do NOT use in the case of head trauma.
To measure – from angle of jaw to nearest nostril.

Oral pharyngeal airway (unconscious and no gag reflex).
To measure – flange aligned to centre of lips, tip to angle of jaw. Insert 'upside down'.

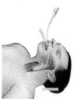

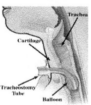

Laryngeal Mask Airway (LMA)

Tracheostomy

➢ Artificial ventilation via bag-valve-mask device.
➢ Endo tracheal intubation.

For management of complete obstruction see choking section.

FIGURE 1.5 Airway management

ADVANCED LIFE SUPPORT (ADULT) ALGORITHM
(RESUCITATION COUNCIL 2015)

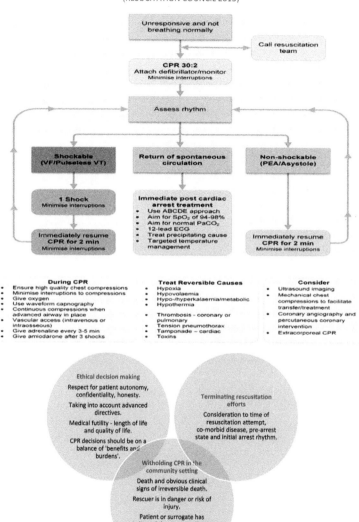

FIGURE 1.6 Advanced life support (adult)

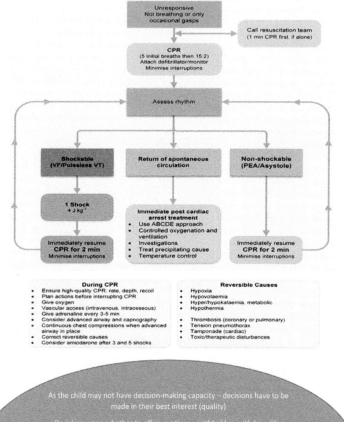

ADVANCED LIFE SUPPORT (PEADIATRIC) ALGORITHM
(RESUCITATION COUNCIL 2015)

Unresponsive
Not breathing or only
occasional gasps

Call resuscitation team
(1 min CPR first, if alone)

CPR
(5 initial breaths then 15:2)
Attach defibrillator/monitor
Minimise interruptions

Assess rhythm

Shockable
(VF/Pulseless VT)

Return of spontaneous
circulation

Non-shockable
(PEA/Asystole)

1 Shock
4 J kg⁻¹

Immediate post cardiac
arrest treatment
• Use ABCDE approach
• Controlled oxygenation and
  ventilation
• Investigations
• Treat precipitating cause
• Temperature control

Immediately resume
CPR for 2 min
Minimise interruptions

Immediately resume
CPR for 2 min
Minimise interruptions

During CPR
• Ensure high-quality CPR: rate, depth, recoil
• Plan actions before interrupting CPR
• Give oxygen
• Vascular access (intravenous, intraosseous)
• Give adrenaline every 3-5 min
• Consider advanced airway and capnography
• Continuous chest compressions when advanced
  airway in place
• Correct reversible causes
• Consider amiodarone after 3 and 5 shocks

Reversible Causes
• Hypoxia
• Hypovolaemia
• Hyper/hypokalaemia, metabolic
• Hypothermia

• Thrombosis (coronary or pulmonary)
• Tension pneumothorax
• Tamponade (cardiac)
• Toxic/therapeutic disturbances

As the child may not have decision-making capacity – decisions have to be
made in their best interest (quality)

Decisions upon whether to offer, continue, withhold or withdraw life-
sustaining interventions will be made.

Issues around futility, preferences (patient/parents), burdens versus benefits
will be considered.

The highest quality and level of communication with everyone involved is
required at all times.

Recommended Summary Plan for Emergency Care and Treatment (ReSPECT)

FIGURE 1.7 Advanced life support (child)

POST RESUSCITATION CARE

Reasons for providing post resuscitation care

The overall aim is to resuscitate as soon as possible and to establish and maintain stable haemodynamic, cardiac and cerebral functions. Depending upon the cause of the cardiac arrest and the severity of the post cardiac arrest syndrome, many patients will require multiple organ support and treatment. Requiring admission to Intensive Care Units.

➢ Reducing risk of recurrence
➢ Preventing further deterioration
➢ Finding the cause of cardiac arrest and treating it
➢ Promoting full recovery of the patient

Post cardiac arrest syndrome is comprised of

- Post cardiac arrest brain injury (e.g. coma, seizures, myoclonus, brain death)
- Post cardiac arrest myocardial dysfunction (hypotension, hypoxaemia)
- Systemic ischaemia/reperfusion response (activation of immune and coagulation pathways leading to multi organ failure and increased risk of infection)
- Persistent precipitating pathology (sepsis, disseminated intravascular coagulation, hyperglycaemia, hypoglycaemia)

Reversible causes of cardiac arrest

The four Hs
1. **Hypoxia** – maximise gas exchange, maximum oxygen during CPR
2. **Hypovolaemia** – fluids to restore intravascular volume
3. **Hypo/hyperkalaemia/ hyperglycaemia/ hypocalcaemia/acidaemia** – calcium chloride IV for hyperkalaemia and hypocalaemia
4. **Hypothermia** – warm slowly (0.5° per hour)

Achievement of return to spontaneous circulation (ROSC) does NOT mean that the patient is out of risk. They will therefore require constant monitoring.

Assess using ABCDE approach. Place patient in recovery position.

Talk to patient to reduce anxiety.

Give 15 litres oxygen via non-rebreathing mask (to maintain oxygen saturation of 94–98% (BTS 2017).

IV access if there is none.

12 lead ECG – cardiac monitoring.

Do not turn the AED off or take defibrillation pads of the patient's chest at any time unless instructed by a doctor.

Continue assessing vital signs.

Ventilation
Hemodynamics
Cardiovascular
Neurological
Metabolic
PCAC

The four Ts
1. **Coronary thrombosis** – diagnosed and treated once return of spontaneous circulation is achieved. Once diagnosed, thrombolysis must be initiated and fibrinolysis for massive pulmonary embolism. Resuscitation attempts should be prolonged for 60–90 minutes after administration (Resuscitation Council 2015).
2. **Tension pneumothorax** – diagnosis is made by symptoms and ultrasound. Treated with emergency needle decompression and chest drain.
3. **Cardiac tamponade** – difficult to diagnose but ultrasound may help. Emergency pericardiocentesis and resuscitative thoracotomy.
4. **Toxins** – revealed by laboratory investigations. Where available appropriate antidotes are used.

Do not attempt cardiopulmonary resuscitation (DNACPR) decisions are common in health care and are concerned with withholding rather than giving treatment. It is seen as a way of protecting patients from harm. Decisions of this nature are made when:

- Patient has capacity to refuse CPR
- CPR is judged very unlikely to be effective (in the case of frailty, co-morbidities)
- When the potential burdens of CPR outweigh the potential benefits

Decisions regarding CPR should be made in the context of the overall care and should involve the patient (when possible) and the next of kin.

FIGURE 1.8 Post-resuscitation care

BASIC LIFE SUPPORT

Safety – Approach with caution – check to see that the scene is safe and there is no danger for yourself or the patient. Where indicated wear Personal Protective Equipment (PPE).

Response – Shout instruction/gently squeeze. Child/infant gently stimulate them. If no response – call for help. If alone, get help/dial 2222 (999 if in community setting). If not alone, send other person to get help/AED.

Airway – Is patient talking? If yes, patent airway clear. If no then open airway (**see below**).

Breathing – Assess for minimum breaths in 10-second period (look/listen/feel – chest movements – adult (2), infants (5) child (3). Be aware of agonal breathing (irregular, slow deep breaths), i.e. patient is not breathing normally.

Circulation – In hospital resuscitation – look for signs of life (response to stimuli/signs of movement). If unresponsive and not breathing normally, start CPR (see below) within 10 seconds (maximum 3 minutes).

Adult BLS

Chest compressions – Heel of dominant hand on lower third of sternum with other hand interlocked, press down 5–6 cm depth (at least 1/3 of chest depth). Rate 100–120 per minute.

30 compressions

Then **2 rescue breaths**

To open airway (head tilt/chin lift) put one hand on forehead to pinch nose and the other to maintain chin lift. Look at chest to see if inflation is successful. Continue with 30 chest compressions to 2 rescue breaths ratio.

As soon as AED arrives, follow instructions.

Modifications

1. Use of pocket mask:

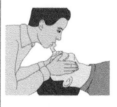

2. If unconscious and breathing effectively, put in recovery position:

Recovery position

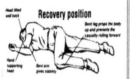

Prevent harm – remove any glasses, watches and jewellery.

Monitor patient's airway very closely for signs of obstruction.

If patient stops breathing then start BLS.

Paediatric BLS

Remove any airway obstruction carefully. For infant, keep head neutral. Do not hyperextend the neck for a child. **Start BLS with 5 rescue breaths** Mouth-to-mouth or mouth-to-nose.

Chest compressions
For an infant under 1 year, locate lower half of sternum and use 2 fingers.

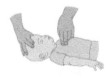

For a child over 1 year, locate lower third of sternum and use 1 or 2 hands.

Press down 1/3 of chest depth at a rate of 100–120 per minute.
15 compressions

Continue with 15 chest compressions to 2 rescue breaths ratio.
If alone do 1 minute of CPR before going for help.

Chain of survival – Key interrelated steps to optimise chances of survival

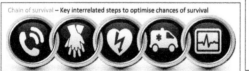

FIGURE 1.9 Early defibrillation

Activity: now test yourself

1 What are the early warning signs of clinical deterioration (there may be more than one)?

a Tachypnoea

b Hypotension

c Tachycardia

d Pallor

e Retraction

2 Answer the following statements with 'True' or 'False'

a Start with five rescue breaths for an adult

b Rate of compressions is 120/min

c If unconscious and not breathing, put in the recovery position

d 30 chest compressions for an adult; 15 compressions for a child

3 List six physiological measures that would indicate patient deterioration

4 Map the symptoms to the correct stage of shock

Stage of shock	Symptoms
Compensatory stage	Slow, laboured breathing, unconscious, multi-organ failure
Progressive stage	Tachycardia, hypotension, tachypnoea, peripheral cyanosis, cool and clammy skin, dizziness
Refractory stage	Increased heart rate, slightly hypotensive or normotensive, pale/clammy skin

5 What is the immediate first aid for wet and dry heat burns?

Answers

1   *Tachypnoea, tachycardia, pallor, retraction*

2   a   False
        Start with five rescue breaths for a child

    b   True
        For both adult and child

    c   False
        Only put in the recovery position if the patient is not breathing and unconscious

    d   True

3   *Respiratory rate, oxygen saturation, systolic blood pressure, heart rate, level of consciousness, temperature*

4   Compensatory – *increased heart rate, slight hypotension or normotensive, pale/clammy skin*
Progressive – *tachycardia, hypotension, tachypnoea, peripheral cyanosis, cool and clammy skin, dizziness*
Refractory – *slow, laboured breathing, unconscious, multi-organ failure*

5   *The aim is to stop the burning process as soon as possible. Leave anything that is stuck into the burnt skin – DO NOT attempt to remove it. Cool burn for 20 minutes under warm running water. Remove clothing/jewellery that is affecting/ will affect the burn. Cover burn with Clingfilm or non-adhesive dressing*

Reflection: ask yourself

1   What do I know now that I did not know before?

2   What I am confused about now?

3   What specific areas do I need to focus on?

4   My action plan for further learning (make objectives SMART: specific, measurable, achievable, realist and timeframe)

CHAPTER 2

Medicines

Sheila Cunningham

Overview

The administration of a medicine is a common but important clinical procedure, and an important aspect of professional practice (NMC 2018b).

Link to *Future Nurse Proficiencies* (NMC 2018a)

Platform 4 Providing and evaluating care: specifically 4.14 and 4.15
Annexe B: Nursing procedures. Section 11: procedural competencies required for best practice, administration of evidence-based medicines and optimisation

Expected knowledge

- Physiology of drug absorption routes, circulation and transportation, and renal function
- Purpose of medicines in care plans

Introduction

The type and manner in which a medicine is administered will determine whether or not the patient gains any clinical benefit, and whether they suffer any adverse effect from their medicines. As the population ages and life expectancy increases, more people are living with several long-term conditions that are being managed with an increasing number of medicines. Problems can arise from other aspects too. These include: drug reactions or non-adherence to medicines will affect the effect of the medicine – between a third and half of prescribed medications for long-term conditions are not used as recommended (Department of Health [DH] 2012); as many as 50% of older people may not be taking their medicines as prescribed (NICE 2012). One of the most common types of adverse events is medication error, which is the most frequent cause of morbidity and preventable death in hospitals (Adams and Koch, 2010). NICE (2015) report that up to 38% of medication errors are serious or fatal, and 42% of those are preventable. Medication errors can take many forms, and may occur at different stages of the medication administration process (from prescription, dispensing or administration) and thus may involve a range of healthcare professionals (prescribers, pharmacists and nurses).

Content

Drug actions in the body	Medication routes and medication formulations	Administering medications safely
Legal aspects of medication administration	Considerations of medications for vulnerable groups	Drug calculations

Learning outcomes

- Discuss the actions of medications on (pharmacodynamics) and travelling through (pharmacokinetics) the human body, explaining desirable and non-desirable effects
- Describe the routes of medication administration and explain safe practice in administering medicines via these routes
- Be familiar with drug calculations (oral and parenteral), including weight and volume conversions
- Explain the legal implications and professional responsibilities of medication administration
- Discuss individual differences and specific issues of safe medication administration for elderly, young and other vulnerable client groups

Key background

Registered healthcare professionals who administer medicines, or an appropriate delegate who administers the medicines, is accountable for their actions, non-actions and omissions, and must exercise professionalism and professional judgement at all times (Royal Pharmaceutical Society 2019). In their new proficiency standards for nurses, the NMC (2018a) indicates that nurses must demonstrate knowledge of pharmacology, understand the principles of safe and effective administration, and the optimisation of medicines, proficiency and accuracy when calculating dosages of prescribed medicines, and be able to apply knowledge of pharmacology to the care of people, demonstrating the ability to progress to a prescribing qualification after registration. They are responsible and accountable – medicines can be dangerous and thus sound knowledge and practice are important to develop and show continually.

The manner in which a medicine is administered will determine, to some extent, whether or not the patient gains any clinical benefit, and whether they suffer any adverse effect from their medicines. The use of powerful and effective drugs, with at times complex drug regimens combined with technological advances, may result in problems. This can result in side effects, challenge of polypharmacy and patient partnership in drug optimisation, as well as medication safety. The term 'medicines optimisation' has replaced 'medicines management' and recognises the active involvement of patients in their medicine therapy. It focuses on actions taken by all health- and social care practitioners and requires greater patient engagement and professional collaboration across health- and social care settings. Nurses administer prescribed medicines and monitor the effects, but also in some areas they are independent prescribers. As indicated by the NMC (2018a) newly qualified nurses will work towards prescribing sooner in their post-registration period, and of course support and supervise other support professionals tasked with administering medicines (e.g. nursing associates).

There are five identifiable phases within the process of medicine administration in which errors may potentially occur: prescription, transcription, dispensing, administering and monitoring patient condition/documenting (Hayes *et al.* 2015). The administration phase is particularly vulnerable to errors; however, simultaneous demands or interruptions during these complex processes increase the likelihood of errors occurring. An earlier systematic review (Keers *et al.* 2013) highlighted that the most commonly reported errors are due to unsafe acts, followed by knowledge-based mistakes and deliberate violations. Error-provoking conditions influencing administration errors include:

- Written communication issues (prescriptions, documentation, transcription) and checking process
- Issues with medicine supply and storage (pharmacy dispensing errors and ward stock management)
- Workload/staff levels and stress levels
- Patient factors (availability, status)
- Interruptions/distractions during drug administration

Nurses have a professional responsibility to safely administer medicines as part of their nursing care, but also to inform, advise and support patients in their care, especially understanding the role of medicines in their treatment or care process.

MEDICINES ADMINISTRATION

The 'RIGHTS'

1. RIGHT Patient
2. RIGHT Medicine
3. RIGHT Dose
4. RIGHT Route
5. RIGHT Time PLUS
6. RIGHT Documentation
7. RIGHT to Refuse

Consider also:

RIGHT Action
RIGHT Form [of medicine]
RIGHT Response

RIGHT Medicine

Proprietary names – are the trade names?
Generic or non-proprietary name is the official accepted name of a drug, as listed in the *British National Formulary (BNF)*.

WHAT IS MEDICINE?

From the Medicines Act 1968:
'A medicine is any substance used for treating, preventing or diagnosing disease, for contraception, for inducing anaesthesia or modifying a normal physiological function'.

According to the MHRA (2017):
'Any substance or combination of substances presented as having properties of preventing or treating disease in human beings'.

RIGHT Route

Oral
Supplied in both solid and liquid forms.
Most common solid forms are *tablets* (tab), *capsules* (cap), and caplets. Liquids are: *elixir, syrup or suspension.*

Parenteral
Intramuscular (IM): into the muscle.
Subcutaneous (SC): into the subcutaneous tissue.
Intravenous (IV): into the vein.
Intradermal (ID): beneath the skin.
Intrathecal (IT): into spinal cavity.

Topical
Cutaneous: applied to the skin.
Transdermal: absorbed through the skin.
Inhalation: breathed into the respiratory tract.
Solutions and ointments: applied to the mucosa of the eyes (optic), nose (nasal), ears (otic) or mouth.
Suppositories or pessaries: applied into body cavities.

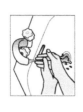

SKILL of ADMINISTRATION – Remember Wash hands BEFORE and AFTER

Prepare necessary equipment – Inform patient of the medication, routes and reasons, and gain consent to administer medication.

RIGHT Patient	RIGHT Medication	RIGHT Time	RIGHT Dose	RIGHT Action	RIGHT Documentation
If elderly/confused or very young Seek verbal confirmation of the patient's name or photo identification.	Prepare **Right Medication** and check **Right Form** for **Right Route** and ensure medicine not expired.	Special requirements? For example, after food.	Administer the medicine. Calculations if needed. Do not leave medicine unattended.	Observe the patient for effects or adverse reactions.	Record that the medicine has been given or not and reasons.

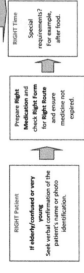

FIGURE 2.1 Medicines administration

DRUG ACTIONS

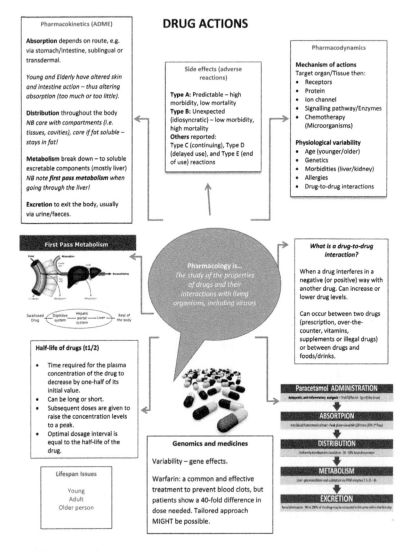

Pharmacokinetics (ADME)

Absorption depends on route, e.g. via stomach/intestine, sublingual or transdermal.

Young and Elderly have altered skin and intestine action – thus altering absorption (too much or too little).

Distribution throughout the body *NB care with compartments (i.e. tissues, cavities), care if fat soluble – stays in fat!*

Metabolism break down – to soluble excretable components (mostly liver) *NB note first pass metabolism when going through the liver!*

Excretion to exit the body, usually via urine/faeces.

Side effects (adverse reactions)

Type A: Predictable – high morbidity, low mortality
Type B: Unexpected (idiosyncratic) – low morbidity, high mortality
Others reported:
Type C (continuing), Type D (delayed use), and Type E (end of use) reactions

Pharmacodynamics

Mechanism of actions
Target organ/Tissue then:
- Receptors
- Protein
- Ion channel
- Signalling pathway/Enzymes
- Chemotherapy (Microorganisms)

Physiological variability
- Age (younger/older)
- Genetics
- Morbidities (liver/kidney)
- Allergies
- Drug-to-drug interactions

First Pass Metabolism

Swallowed Drug → Digestive system → Hepatic portal system → Liver → Rest of the body

Pharmacology is... The study of the properties of drugs and their interactions with living organisms, including viruses

What is a drug-to-drug interaction?

When a drug interferes in a negative (or positive) way with another drug. Can increase or lower drug levels.

Can occur between two drugs (prescription, over-the-counter, vitamins, supplements or illegal drugs) or between drugs and foods/drinks.

Half-life of drugs (t1/2)

- Time required for the plasma concentration of the drug to decrease by one-half of its initial value.
- Can be long or short.
- Subsequent doses are given to raise the concentration levels to a peak.
- Optimal dosage interval is equal to the half-life of the drug.

Lifespan Issues

Young
Adult
Older person

Genomics and medicines

Variability – gene effects.

Warfarin: a common and effective treatment to prevent blood clots, but patients show a 40-fold difference in dose needed. Tailored approach MIGHT be possible.

Paracetamol ADMINISTRATION

ABSORPTION

DISTRIBUTION

METABOLISM

EXCRETION

FIGURE 2.2 Drug actions

NON-MEDICAL PRESCRIBING

Legal aspects to consider

Medicines Act (1968)
Misuse of Drugs Regulations (2001)
Royal Pharmaceutical Society Competency Framework (RPS 2016)

Skills needed to prescribe

- Clinical knowledge and skills
- Clinical experience
- Pharmacology knowledge
- Knowledge of legislation and regulatory frameworks
- Local policies and guidance

Prescribe safely: 3 domains

1. Consultation and knowledge
2. Prescribe effectively
3. Prescribe in Context

What is a non-medical prescriber?

Non-medical prescribing, is undertaken by a health professional who is not a doctor, e.g. nurses, pharmacists and other health professionals who prescribe are highly skilled in their specialist area.

Three nurse/midwife types:

- Community Practitioner Nurse Prescribers (CPNP) prescribe formulary contains appliances, dressings, pharmacy (P), general sales list (GSL) and thirteen prescription only medicines (POMs).
- Nurse Independent Prescribers (NIP) may prescribe medicines and products listed in the BNF, unlicensed medicines and all controlled drugs in schedules 2–5.
- Supplementary Nurse Prescribers.

PRESCRIPTION WRITING

Prescriptions must:

- be legible
- be legal
- be signed
- use approved names of drugs
- use clear units and route
- not use abbreviations
- be careful with decimal points
- include all information for safe administration.

Minimising errors

- Consultation: appropriateness of medication (type, effect)
- Prescription writing (names, legibility, abbreviations, units)
- Care with special groups (elderly, very young), chronic complex morbidities.

Prescribing Governance

- Prescribe safely
- Prescribe professionally (codes/law)
- Reflect to improve prescribing practice
- Prescribe as part of a team

The Consultation

- Assess the patient
- Consider the options
- Reach a shared (with other professionals) decision
- Prescribe
- Provide information
- Monitor and review

PRINCIPLES of PRESCRIBING

Resources

- eMedicines compendium
- Local pharmacy/pharmacist British National Formulary
- Electronic prescribing service

FIGURE 2.3 Non-medical prescribing

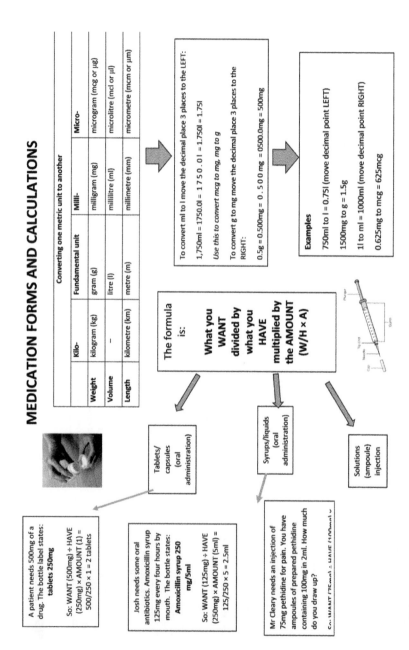

FIGURE 2.4 Medication forms and calculations

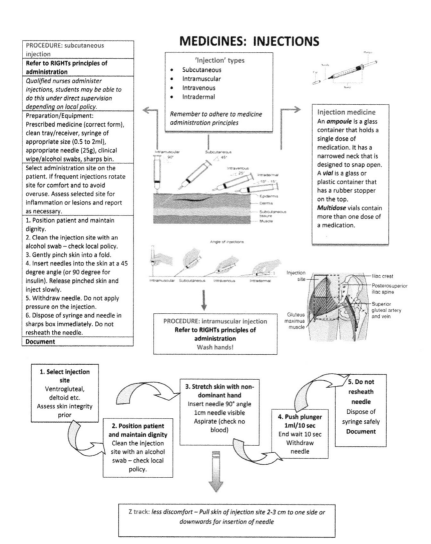

FIGURE 2.5 Injections

Activity: now test yourself

1 In relation to medicine administration, which of these are correct (there is more than one)?

   a   Right dose

   b   Right patient

   c   Right environment

   d   Right route

   e   Right documentation

2 How can a nurse check a patient's identity to give a medicine if they cannot communicate?

   a   Fingerprints

   b   Ask a relative or friend to confirm their identity

   c   Use a photographic record of their identity attached to documents

   d   Ask the admitting or charge nurse

3 Medications subject to *first-pass metabolism* are affected by which route of administration?

   a   Oral

   b   Intravenous

   c   Rectal

   d   Subcutaneous

4 Type B drug interactions refer to:

   a   Predictable adverse effects with low mortality but high morbidity

   b   Unpredictable: adverse reactions with low morbidity and mortality c   Predictable adverse effects with high mortality

d   Unpredictable adverse effects with high mortality but low morbidity

5   List three errors in drug prescription writing that may be dangerous.

Answers

1 a, b, d, e
   Although the environment is important medications can be given in a variety of environments, but the same principles of safety apply whatever the environment – none is 'right'.

2 c
   Concrete tangible evidence of identity is needed; the NMC (2007) and Royal Pharmaceutical Society (2019) suggest evidence such as photographic ID.

3 a
   Oral medications are absorbed by the gastrointestinal tract, and from there go to the liver via the portal hepatic vein. It is in the liver that enzymes begin the breakdown of the drugs (or first-pass metabolism), with the remaining medication termed its 'bioavailability'.

4 d
   Adverse drug reactions (ADRs) are increasingly common and are a significant cause of morbidity and mortality. Historically, ADRs have been classified as type A or B. Type A reactions are predictable from the known pharmacology of a drug and associated with high morbidity and low mortality. Type B reactions are idiosyncratic, bizarre or novel responses that cannot be predicted from the known pharmacology of a drug, and are associated with low morbidity and high mortality. Nurses and other healthcare personnel are required to report ADRs through the Yellow Card Scheme.

5 May include: *not legible, abbreviations, decimal points, unclear route, not signed, no approved name.*

Reflection: ask yourself

1 What do I know now that I didn't know before?

2 What am I confused/unclear about?

3 What areas do I need to focus on?

4 My action plan for further learning (make objectives SMART)

CHAPTER 3

Infection control

Sheila Cunningham

Overview

The NMC (2018a) in their recently produced standards of nurse proficiency indicate that nurses must: *'protect health through understanding and applying the principles of infection prevention and control, including communicable disease surveillance and antimicrobial stewardship and resistance'* (NMC, 2018a: 12, Section 2.12). It is thus a key skill that must be developed and practised regularly for reduction of infection risk, which affects patients, carers and healthcare professionals, as a priority.

Link to Future Nurse Proficiencies (NMC 2018a)

Platform 2 Promoting health and preventing ill health: specifically 2.12: protect health through understanding and applying the principles of infection prevention and control, including communicable disease surveillance and antimicrobial stewardship and resistance.)

Annexe B: Nursing procedures Section 9: use evidence-based, best practice approaches to meet needs for care and support for the prevention and management of infection, accurately assessing the person's capacity for independence and self-care, and initiating appropriate interventions

Expected knowledge

- The difference among viruses, bacteria and fungi
- What is meant by 'drug-resistant microbes'?
- The role of commensal organisms

Introduction

The prevalence of healthcare-associated infections in hospitals in England in 2016 was 6.4%. The most common types of healthcare-associated infection are respiratory infections (including pneumonia and infections of the lower respiratory tract; 22.8%), urinary tract infections (17.2%) and surgical site infections (15.7%) (NICE 2014; Public Health England, 2018). This highlights the need for all healthcare professionals to engage in infection control approaches to minimise serious consequences for patients and clients. .

Content

Infection cycle	Microorganisms and pathophysiology	Handwashing
Isolation	Healthcare-acquired infections	Waste disposal

Learning outcomes

- Outline the transmission of infection, the risks and potential consequences to the patients across the lifespan and the range of organisms involved
- Analyse the processes and practices of standard precautions and the use of isolation and personal protective equipment to minimise healthcare-associated infections
- Explain and critically appraise the healthcare environment waste risk and appropriate waste disposal, or their management to minimise overall risk
- Explain the necessity of practices associated with effective hand hygiene
- Explain the principles and procedures of standard isolation techniques for patients with infectious disease or who are immunocompromised and vulnerable to infectious disease

Key background

Infectious microorganisms occur naturally in the environment, potentially causing harm, but can also be introduced to patients and clients through the caring practices of and encounters with healthcare professionals. Healthcare-associated infections (HCAIs) arise across a wide range of clinical conditions and can affect people of all ages. HCAI is a catch-all term for a wide range of infections that can exacerbate existing or underlying conditions, delay recovery and adversely affect quality of life. The most well-known HCAIs include those caused by meticillin-resistant *Staphylococcus aureus* (MRSA), meticillin-sensitive *S. aureus* (MSSA), *Clostridium difficile* (*C. difficile*) and *Escherichia coli* (*E. coli*). Public Health bodies and all UK countries collect data and monitor trends regularly for the UK. It is estimated that 300,000 patients a year in England acquire a HCAI as a result of care within the NHS.

The NMC (2018a: 36), in their future nurse standard, indicates that it is a key role for nurses to '*observe, assess and respond rapidly to potential infection risks using best practice guidelines*' (standard 9.1). This is then expanded to the wider public health sphere by moving beyond applying the principles of infection prevention and control to the skill of communicable disease surveillance (or outbreak and spread patterns), and antimicrobial stewardship and resistance, to minimise the issue of 'superbugs' or microbial drug resistance.

INFECTION CYCLE AND CONTROL

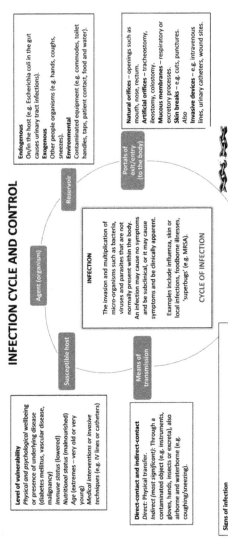

Level of vulnerability
Physical and psychological wellbeing or presence of underlying disease (diabetes mellitus, vascular disease, malignancy)
Immune status (lowered)
Nutritional status (malnourished)
Age (extremes – very old or very young)
Medical interventions or invasive techniques (e.g. IV lines or catheters)

Endogenous
On/in the host (e.g. Escherichia coli in the gut causes urinary tract infections).
Exogenous
Other people organisms (e.g. hands, coughs, sneezes).
Environmental
Contaminated equipment (e.g. commodes, toilet handles, taps, patient contact, food and water).

Natural orifices – openings such as mouth, nose, rectum.
Artificial orifices – tracheostomy, ileostomy, colostomy.
Mucous membranes – respiratory or excretory processes.
Skin breaks – e.g. cuts, punctures.
Also
Invasive devices – e.g. intravenous lines, urinary catheters, wound sites.

Reservoir

Agent (organism)

Portals of exit/entry (to the body)

Susceptible host

Means of transmission

INFECTION

The invasion and multiplication of micro-organisms such as bacteria, viruses and parasites that are not normally present within the body.
An infection may cause no symptoms and be subclinical, or it may cause symptoms and be clinically apparent.

Examples include influenza, skin or local infections, foodborne illnesses, 'superbugs' (e.g. MRSA).

CYCLE OF INFECTION

Direct-contact and indirect-contact
Direct: Physical transfer.
Indirect (most significant): Through a contaminated object (e.g. instruments, gloves, hands, insects or excreta), also airborne and waterborne (e.g. coughing/sneezing).

Break cycle of infection
Safe working practices involve:
- effective hand hygiene
- standard universal precautions (of blood and body fluids)
- effective cleaning, disinfection or sterilisation
- aseptic technique
- safe disposal of waste, non-reusable instruments, sharps and linen
- isolation precautions, if patients have known or suspected infection.

Signs of infection
Signs and symptoms of a bacterial infection vary depending on the location of the infection and the type of bacteria causing it.
However, some general symptoms of a bacterial infection include:
- fever
- feeling tired or fatigued
- swollen lymph nodes in the neck, armpits or groin
- headache
- nausea or vomiting
For wounds, observe for redness, heat, pain, swelling and loss of

FIGURE 3.1 Infection cycle and control

HAND HYGIENE

Hand hygiene procedure

Six steps (WHO 2009):
- Wet your hands with water (warm or cold).
- Apply enough soap to cover the hands and lather. Alcohol-based handrub can be used if immediate access to soap and water is unavailable.
1. Rub hands palm-to-palm.
2. Rub the back of the left hand with the right palm using interlaced fingers. Repeat with the other hand.
3. Rub palms together with fingers interlaced.
4. Rub the backs of the fingers against the palms with fingers interlocked.
5. Clasp the left thumb with the right hand and rub in rotation. Repeat reversing the hands.
6. Rub in a circular motion the palm with the tips of the fingers. Repeat with the other hand.
- Rinse hands with water (warm or cold).
- Dry thoroughly, ideally with a disposable towel.
- Use the disposable towel to turn off the tap and discard towel.

Nurses are advised not to wear artificial fingernails or extenders when in direct contact with patients and to keep natural nails short.

What is hand hygiene?

WHO (2009: 7) define it as:
Any action of hygienic hand antisepsis in order to reduce transient microbial flora (generally performed either by handrubbing with an alcohol-based formulation or handwashing with plain or antimicrobial soap and water).

Rationale
Health care workers have the greatest potential to spread micro-organisms that may result in infection due to the number of times they have contact with patients or the patient environment.

Hands are therefore a very efficient vehicle for transferring micro-organisms.

The term hand hygiene includes handwashing, surgical scrub and the use of alcohol gel. The type of hand hygiene is dependent on the type of care to be carried out.

When to wash hands

RCN (2018) recommend several points to performing hand hygiene, including:
- Attending to direct patient care
- Switching between patients
- Before putting on personal protective equipment and after taking it off
- Before giving the patient/client food or drinks
- After making the patient's/client's bed
- After helping the patient/client back from the toilet
- After removing any waste from the patient's/client's living area
- Before eating
- When handling raw food
- After using the toilet
- After coughing or sneezing
- After using a disposable tissue
- When starting and finishing work

Glove awareness
Gloves are not a substitute for hand hygiene. It can lead to irritability, skin sensitivity and in some cases dermatitis. To minimise this risk ensure these procedures are followed:
- Wet hands well before applying soap.
- Wash hands with soap and water when visibly dirty or soiled with blood or other body fluids.
- Wash hands with soap and water where alcohol handrubs are less effective, e.g. patients with known or suspected infections.
- Wash hands with soap and water if alcohol-based handrub is not available. Hand wipes may be helpful in community settings.
- Use an alcohol-based handrub as routine hand hygiene in all other clinical situations.
  (Adapted from WHO 2009)

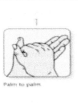
1 Palm to palm.

2 Right palm over left dorsum and left palm over right dorsum.

3 Palm to palm, fingers interlaced.

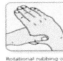
4 Backs of fingers to opposing palms with fingers interlocked.

5 Rotational rubbing of right thumb clasped in left palm, then vice versa.

6 Rotational rubbing, backwards and forwards with clasped fingers of hand in left palm, then vice versa.

FIGURE 3.2 Hand hygiene

HOW MICROBES CAUSE DISEASE/ILLNESS

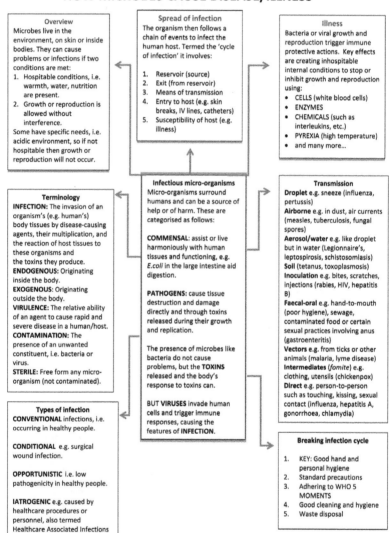

Overview
Microbes live in the environment, on skin or inside bodies. They can cause problems or infections if two conditions are met:
1. Hospitable conditions, i.e. warmth, water, nutrition are present.
2. Growth or reproduction is allowed without interference.
Some have specific needs, i.e. acidic environment, so if not hospitable then growth or reproduction will not occur.

Spread of infection
The organism then follows a chain of events to infect the human host. Termed the 'cycle of infection' it involves:

1. Reservoir (source)
2. Exit (from reservoir)
3. Means of transmission
4. Entry to host (e.g. skin breaks, IV lines, catheters)
5. Susceptibility of host (e.g. illness)

Illness
Bacteria or viral growth and reproduction trigger immune protective actions. Key effects are creating inhospitable internal conditions to stop or inhibit growth and reproduction using:
- CELLS (white blood cells)
- ENZYMES
- CHEMICALS (such as interleukins, etc.)
- PYREXIA (high temperature)
- and many more...

Terminology
INFECTION: The invasion of an organism's (e.g. human's) body tissues by disease-causing agents, their multiplication, and the reaction of host tissues to these organisms and the toxins they produce.
ENDOGENOUS: Originating inside the body.
EXOGENOUS: Originating outside the body.
VIRULENCE: The relative ability of an agent to cause rapid and severe disease in a human/host.
CONTAMINATION: The presence of an unwanted constituent, i.e. bacteria or virus.
STERILE: Free form any micro-organism (not contaminated).

Infectious micro-organisms
Micro-organisms surround humans and can be a source of help or of harm. These are categorised as follows:

COMMENSAL: assist or live harmoniously with human tissues and functioning, e.g. *E.coli* in the large intestine aid digestion.

PATHOGENS: cause tissue destruction and damage directly and through toxins released during their growth and replication.

The presence of microbes like bacteria do not cause problems, but the **TOXINS** released and the body's response to toxins can.

BUT **VIRUSES** invade human cells and trigger immune responses, causing the features of **INFECTION**.

Transmission
Droplet e.g. sneeze (influenza, pertussis)
Airborne e.g. in dust, air currents (measles, tuberculosis, fungal spores)
Aerosol/water e.g. like droplet but in water (Legionnaire's, leptospirosis, schistosomiasis)
Soil (tetanus, toxoplasmosis)
Inoculation e.g. bites, scratches, injections (rabies, HIV, hepatitis B)
Faecal-oral e.g. hand-to-mouth (poor hygiene), sewage, contaminated food or certain sexual practices involving anus (gastroenteritis)
Vectors e.g. from ticks or other animals (malaria, lyme disease)
Intermediates (*fomite*) e.g. clothing, utensils (chickenpox)
Direct e.g. person-to-person such as touching, kissing, sexual contact (influenza, hepatitis A, gonorrhoea, chlamydia)

Types of infection
CONVENTIONAL infections, i.e. occurring in healthy people.

CONDITIONAL e.g. surgical wound infection.

OPPORTUNISTIC i.e. low pathogenicity in healthy people.

IATROGENIC e.g. caused by healthcare procedures or personnel, also termed Healthcare Associated Infections (HCAI).

Breaking infection cycle

1. KEY: Good hand and personal hygiene
2. Standard precautions
3. Adhering to WHO 5 MOMENTS
4. Good cleaning and hygiene
5. Waste disposal

FIGURE 3.3 How microbes cause disease/illness

CURRENT UK VACCINATION SCHEDULE (NHS 2016)

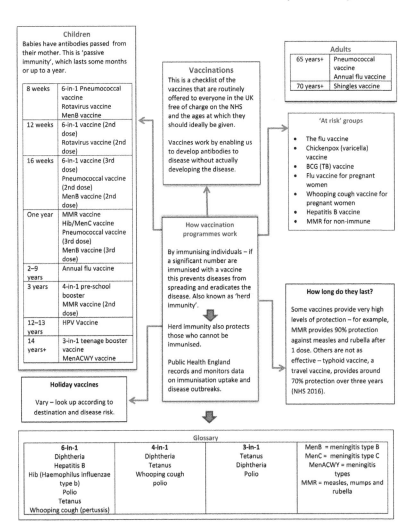

Children

Babies have antibodies passed from their mother. This is 'passive immunity', which lasts some months or up to a year.

8 weeks	6-in-1 Pneumococcal vaccine Rotavirus vaccine MenB vaccine
12 weeks	6-in-1 vaccine (2nd dose) Rotavirus vaccine (2nd dose)
16 weeks	6-in-1 vaccine (3rd dose) Pneumococcal vaccine (2nd dose) MenB vaccine (2nd dose)
One year	MMR vaccine Hib/MenC vaccine Pneumococcal vaccine (3rd dose) MenB vaccine (3rd dose)
2–9 years	Annual flu vaccine
3 years	4-in-1 pre-school booster MMR vaccine (2nd dose)
12–13 years	HPV Vaccine
14 years+	3-in-1 teenage booster vaccine MenACWY vaccine

Holiday vaccines

Vary – look up according to destination and disease risk.

Vaccinations

This is a checklist of the vaccines that are routinely offered to everyone in the UK free of charge on the NHS and the ages at which they should ideally be given.

Vaccines work by enabling us to develop antibodies to disease without actually developing the disease.

How vaccination programmes work

By immunising individuals – if a significant number are immunised with a vaccine this prevents diseases from spreading and eradicates the disease. Also known as 'herd immunity'.

Herd immunity also protects those who cannot be immunised.

Public Health England records and monitors data on immunisation uptake and disease outbreaks.

Adults

65 years+	Pneumococcal vaccine Annual flu vaccine
70 years+	Shingles vaccine

'At risk' groups

- The flu vaccine
- Chickenpox (varicella) vaccine
- BCG (TB) vaccine
- Flu vaccine for pregnant women
- Whooping cough vaccine for pregnant women
- Hepatitis B vaccine
- MMR for non-immune

How long do they last?

Some vaccines provide very high levels of protection – for example, MMR provides 90% protection against measles and rubella after 1 dose. Others are not as effective – typhoid vaccine, a travel vaccine, provides around 70% protection over three years (NHS 2016).

Glossary			
6-in-1 Diphtheria Hepatitis B Hib (Haemophilus influenzae type b) Polio Tetanus Whooping cough (pertussis)	**4-in-1** Diphtheria Tetanus Whooping cough polio	**3-in-1** Tetanus Diphtheria Polio	MenB = meningitis type B MenC = meningitis type C MenACWY = meningitis types MMR = measles, mumps and rubella

FIGURE 3.4 Current UK vaccination schedule

IMMUNE SYSTEM /INFLAMMATION

Overview

The immune system is a host defence system comprising many biological structures (cells and tissues) and processes (recognition and attack) within an organism that protects against disease.
Organisms include bacteria, viruses and funghi (see Figure 3.3).

Immunity is:
- resistance to microbial attacks
- protection and defence in the longer term.

Types of immunity

1. Innate (natural, inbuilt) and *non-specific*
   a. External (barriers)
   b. Internal defences

2. Acquired/active (body response to an antigen) and *specific*
   a. Active
   b. Passive

Innate – *barriers*

Physical:
- Skin
- Mucus
- Nasal hair
- Cilia

Chemical:
- Phagocytes
- Inflammation
- Fever
- Interferons
- Complement system
- Natural killer cells

Acquired/active immunity

Active: contact with antigen
Memory
- T cells – various types
- B cells – antibodies
- Antigen presenting cells (e.g. macrophages)

Passive:
No memory
- Antibodies from another source, e.g. mother, donor
- Short-term protection

Excessive immune response
- Allergic response
- Hypersensitivity

Vaccines/immunisations

- A vaccine is a biological preparation that provides active acquired immunity to a particular disease.
- A vaccine typically contains an agent that resembles a disease-causing micro-organism and is often made from weakened or killed forms of the microbe, its toxins, or one of its surface proteins.

Inflammatory response

Fever
- Fever is also known as pyrexia and febrile response.
- Body temperature above the normal range due to an increase in the body's temperature set point (between 37.5 and 38.3°C).
- Patient may feel hot and sweaty or have muscle contractions and a feeling of cold.
- May trigger a febrile seizure in young children.

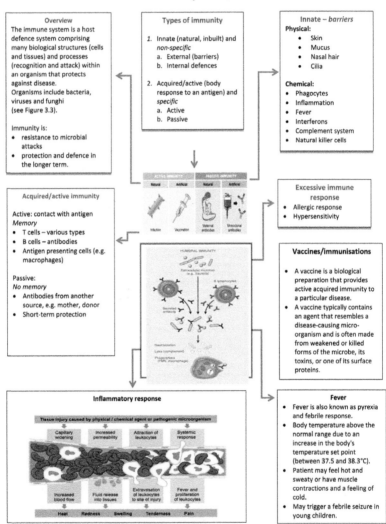

FIGURE 3.5 Immune system/inflammation

STANDARD PRECAUTIONS AND WASTE DISPOSAL

Isolation nursing

Isolation nursing is the use of infection control practices aimed at controlling the spread of, and eradicating, pathogenic organisms.
May be in the patient's own room or home.

STANDARD PRECAUTIONS

These measures must always be provided during patient care with exposure to potentially infected material such as bodily fluids, blood etc.

Components:
1. Handwashing
2. Barrier precautions/PPE
3. Sharps disposal
4. Handling of contaminated material

Waste disposal
- Clinical and non-clinical waste
- Sorting not advised (dangerous)
- Use of colour-coded bags (not filled more than three quarters full, tied securely and appropriately labelled)
- Clinical waste categorised according to level of risk, e.g.
  - yellow/orange bags: clinical waste – infectious waste/body fluids etc. (for incineration)
  - black/clear bags: non-infectious, non-sharps
  - red: highly infected dressings, soiled waste (for incineration)
  - sharps boxes: for needles, cannulae, etc. (rigid containers)

Practical considerations

Preparation:
- Explain the need for isolation and gain consent.
- Decontaminate hands.
- Single room / group area.
- Physical separation (closed doors).
- Appropriate colour-coded isolation precaution sign.
- Appropriate PPE.
- Specifically designated equipment, e.g. sphygmomanometers, thermometers, commodes etc.
- Maintain confidentiality.

During:
- Limit the number of staff.
- Psychological needs of the patient during isolation.
- PPE – as appropriate.
- Wash and dry hands thoroughly after removing protective clothing and before leaving the isolation room.
- Dispose of all excreta promptly.
- All linen must be placed into water-soluble alginate bags.
- Deal with any blood/body fluid spillage immediately.
- Follow Infection Control Team's/advisors' advice on cleaning.
- Minimal movements between departments/clinics is advised.
- All staff and visitors to adhere to PPE and hand hygiene.
- Documents and charts kept outside the patient's room.

Following (end of isolation):
- Enhanced cleaning of isolated area/equipment according to local policy.

Accidents or incidents

Spillage must be cleaned up immediately.

Mercury, toxic products

⬇

SPILLAGE KIT

⬇

No KIT?

⬇

Use disinfection products (check local policy) then wipe up with disposable cloths and dispose of in a clinical waste (yellow/red) bag.

Sharps disposal

Includes hypodermic, suture or biopsy needles, razor or scalpel blades, broken glass or other sharp objects.
- Never re-sheath needles.
- Practise a safe-handling technique, do not pass sharps from hand to hand – use a neutral zone (tray).
- Dispose of sharps into sharps box immediately after use.
- Do not overfill sharps box (maximum ¾ full then sealed prior to disposal).

What precautions to take?

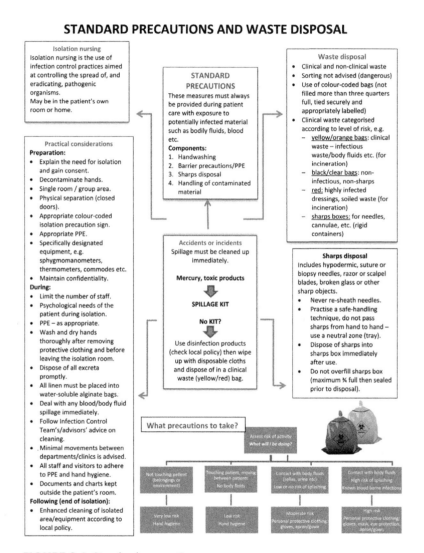

FIGURE 3.6 Standard precautions

ISOLATION AND PROTECTIVE PROCESSES

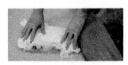

Gloves

- Protect hands from becoming contaminated with organic matter and micro-organisms.
- Prevent the transfer of organisms already on the skin.

Gloves are for invasive procedures, by those who have cuts or grazes. All activities that have a risk of exposure to blood, body fluids, secretions and excretions, and when handling sharps and contaminated instruments. Gloves are not appropriate for routine care practices (assisting with meals, bathing etc.) and not as a substitute for adequate hand hygiene.

Isolation

- Prevent transfer of infection from the patient to others (source isolation).
- Prevent transfer of infection to another susceptible person (protective isolation).

In general:
- Single room (if possible)
- Use of PPE
- Single-use equipment
- Dispose of spillages/body fluids carefully
- Limit visitors/persons entering room
- Maintain patient confidentiality

Spillages

Blood spillages must be cleaned as soon as they occur in order to prevent unnecessary exposure. Suitable protective clothing should be worn: gloves, aprons etc.

Spillage kits are often available, e.g. for dangerous products like mercury (*COSHH*, HSE 2002). If no spillage kits are provided for bodily fluid spills the preferred method for cleaning up spillages is use of disinfection products (as identified in local policy) then wiped up with disposable cloths and disposed of in a clinical waste (yellow or orange) bag.

PPE: varied
Minimum aprons and gloves
- White – where there is the risk of contamination from blood and body fluids.
- Yellow – when caring for patients in isolation.
- Green – when handling and serving food.

How to put on sterile gloves:

- Wash hands
- Check glove package for integrity and expiry date
- Sterile gloves are packaged pre-cuffed
- Set up your 'sterile field' on a clean dressing trolley
- Open and empty contents onto the sterile towel
- Only touch the inner aspect of the cuff
- Using dominant hand to secure the glove, slide the non-dominant hand into the glove
- Put the second glove on, only touching the outer aspect of the glove with your sterile gloved hand
- Sterile gloves should not come into contact with non-sterile surfaces or objects

Personal protective equipment (PPE)
Putting it on:
- Gown
- Mask
- Googles
- Gloves

Removal:
- Avoid contamination at all steps
- Peel off gown and gloves and roll inside together – dispose of them safely
- Wash hands
- Remove googles/face shield/mask from behind and dispose of safely
- Wash hands

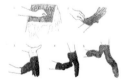

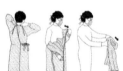

FIGURE 3.7 Isolation and protective processes

Activity: now test yourself

Multiple-choice questions

1   One of the most important aspects of infection protection and control is:

    a   Washing your hands with antibacterial soap

    b   Not allowing hair to fall below your collar line

    c   Use of gloves when washing patients

    d   Good regular hand hygiene

2   Infections caused by or associated with treatments people receive are known as:

    a   Hospital-induced infections

    b   Care negligence infections

    c   Iatrogenic infections

    d   Opportunistic environment-associated infections

3   Aseptic technique refers to:

    a   Any procedure involving gloves

    b   Any procedure performed under sterile conditions

    c   Any procedure involving surgery

    d   Any procedure involving blood or body fluids

4   Standard precautions are used only when:

    a   Caring for patients with highly transmissible infections

    b   Carrying out procedures that involve sharps and body fluids

    c   Patients with infections are in isolation

    d   caring for all patients at all times

5   Which of the following is NOT correct with regard to the inflammatory response?

   a   Damaged cells release T cells, which are the body's own antibiotics to fight the injury or infection.

   b   It occurs when tissues are injured by bacteria, trauma, toxins, heat or any other cause.

   c   Damaged cells release chemicals including histamine, bradykinin and prostaglandins.

   d   Chemicals cause increased blood flow, heat, swelling and pain to the injured area

   e   Pus is formed after phagocytosis of dead tissue, dead bacteria, and live and dead phagocytes.

Application challenge

Label the following **YES** if you think non-sterile gloves are necessary and **NO** if you think they are not. If unsure, read the concept maps again (Figures 3.1–3.7).

1 Administering a nasogastric feed:	**YES/NO**
2 Taking a blood pressure postoperatively	**YES/NO**
3 Changing a catheter bag	**YES/NO**
4 Making a bed	**YES/NO**
5 Giving a patient a suppository	**YES/NO**
6 Bed bathing an uninfected patient	**YES/NO**
7 Giving a patient a drink	**YES/NO**
8 Taking blood samples	**YES/NO**

Answers

1 d

> The national epic3 guidelines indicate that hand washing is one of the main core principles for preventing healthcare-associated infections in hospital or any other healthcare settings (Loveday et al. 2014). So long as the three stages are followed (preparation, washing and drying), it is good practice for washing to last a minimum of 15 seconds. Antibacterial soap is not required. Alcohol gel may also be used.

2 b

> Iatrogenic refers to the consequences of healthcare personal interventions or actions. It is quite an old term; however, it is not only used for infections. It is also known as healthcare associated infection.

3 d

> Aseptic technique means 'without microorganisms'. Aseptic technique refers to the procedure used to avoid the introduction of pathogenic organisms into a vulnerable body site or invasive device. The principal aim of an aseptic technique is to protect the patient from contamination by pathogenic organisms during medical and nursing procedures. Aseptic non-touch technique (ANTT) is the practice of avoiding contamination by not touching key elements such as the tip of a needle, the seal of an intravenous connector after it has been decontaminated or the inside surface of a sterile dressing where it will be in contact with the wound

4 a

> Revisiting the processes in inflammation it is clear that it is a protective response resulting in redness (cell damage, chemicals and blood flow), heat (cell damage, chemicals and blood flow), pain (due to local chemicals such as histamine), swelling (chemicals and increased blood flow, invasion by phagocytes) and potentially loss of function. The role of T cells comes in later if this is an infection and an extension of the inflammatory response, but is not part of it initially.

5

Application challenge

YES = 1, 3, 5
NO = 2, 4, 6, 7, 8

Note that 8 is a trick – this ought to be sterile gloves

Reflection: ask yourself

1 What do I know now that I didn't know before?

2 What am I confused/unclear about?

3 What areas do I need to focus on?

4 My action plan for further learning (make objectives SMART)

CHAPTER 4

Skin and wounds

Sheila Cunningham and Tina Moore

Overview

Patients requiring wound care can be found in the community, secondary care and long-term care institutions, and range from infants to elderly people. The annual cost incurred by the NHS in managing wounds and associated comorbidities was estimated to be £5.3 billion. This equated to 4% of the total expenditure by the NHS in the UK (Guest *et al.* 2017).

Link to *Future Nurse Proficiencies* (NMC 2018a)

Platform 4 Providing and evaluating care.
Specifically 2.12

To protect health through understanding and applying the principles of infection prevention and control, including communicable disease surveillance and antimicrobial stewardship and resistance.
Annexe B: Nursing procedures Section 4: use evidence-based, best practice approaches for meeting the needs for care and support with hygiene and the maintenance of skin integrity, accurately assessing the person's capacity for independence and self-care and initiating appropriate interventions

Expected knowledge

- Skin tissue composition
- Role of the skin in homeostasis and protection
- Normal healing

Introduction

A 'wound' can be defined as a break or lack of continuity in the epithelial covering of the human body. Wounds can be classified in various ways. All aspects of skin and soft-tissue wounds, including acute surgical wounds, pressure ulcers and all forms of leg ulceration, are encompassed in the specialty of tissue viability. Wound care can be a challenging and complex area of practice, and nurses must take individual responsibility for updating their knowledge, skills and ongoing competence.

Content

Skin integrity and healing process	Wound types	Aseptic non-touch technique (ANTT)
Sutures and clips	Bandaging	Wound swabs

Learning outcomes

- Discuss the wound-healing processes and factors that affect a patient's ability to heal
- Explain the principles of wound assessment and wound-care management plan, and challenges across the lifespan and care environments
- Rationalise when and how to undertake an aseptic technique
- Demonstrate through description how to remove sutures and clips
- Explain the principles of bandaging techniques

Key background

Wound healing is the collective term for the physiological process that repairs and restores damage to the skin. It is a complex process that relies on a number of interrelated factors. The same basic cellular and biochemical processes are involved in the healing process of all wounds independent of type. A wound by definition is a breakdown in the protective function of the skin: the loss of continuity of epithelium, with or without loss of underlying connective tissue (i.e. muscle, bone, nerves). This may follow injury to the skin or underlying tissues caused by surgery, a cut, chemicals, heat/cold, or friction/shearing forces, pressure or a result of disease, such as leg ulcers or tumours. It is estimated that more than 2.2 million people over the age of 18 years were managed in the NHS in 2013–2014. Of these, 89% were acute wounds, 58% chronic wounds and 87% of unspecified wound type, with a prevalence across all categories estimated to be growing at around 11% per year (Guest *et al.* 2017). This is a tremendous burden on resources and healthcare personnel.

The NMC (2018a), in their document *Future Nurse Proficiencies*, indicates that nurses are pivotal in knowing and using evidence-based, best practice approaches to meet the needs for care and support with hygiene and the maintenance of skin integrity. Furthermore they state, in Standard 4.6, that nurses ought to possess the skills of using aseptic techniques when managing wound and drainage processes. Wounds are not confined to one specific group of patients, but may occur in any. Children and young people may experience severe wounds from a variety of causes and need the same principles of care in an age-appropriate way. Similarly, social and behavioural activities, such as being homeless, drug taking and generally poor physical condition, may result in a wound that requires careful approaches, especially when dealing with confused or disoriented patients or clients. As in any nursing activity, this is holistic and patient centred, and the principles are applied appropriately.

SKIN AND HYGIENE

Thermoregulation

Hot
Peripheral temperature receptors (PTR) in the skin stimulate hypothalamus to send signals to parasympathetic nervous system, leading to vasodilation directing warm blood from core organs to the skin. Heat loss through radiation and conduction is increased. Production of sweat through sweat glands.

Cold
PTR stimulate hypothalamus to send signals to the sympathetic nervous system causing vasoconstriction (decreasing blood flow to skin) preventing heat loss. Shivering occurs to produce heat. Blood is redirected to vital organs.

Functions of the skin

- Protection, acting as a physical barrier to infection and injury. It is the body's first line of defence against infection.
- Maintaining body temperature.
- Secretion of sebum.
- Receiving stimuli.
- Excretion of water, salts and several organic compounds.
- Vitamin D synthesis.

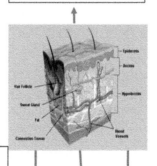

Skill: washing a patient

1. **Preparation**
- Explain procedure and gain valid consent.
- Remove bedding covers, keeping top sheet on patient. Undress patient maintaining privacy and dignity.
2. **Face and neck**
- Place first towel on chest.
- Wash face and neck area. Avoid soap/cleanser getting into eyes. Let patient do this if able.
- Pat dry with second towel.

3. **Upper body**
- Includes arms and chest. Wash arm furthest away first. Rinse off soap and pat dry with towel.
- Sit patient forward and repeat for the back.
- Replace patient's top clothing.

4. **Lower body**
- Wash both legs and feet, one at a time.
- Change water then was the genital area (let patient do this themselves if able). Then was the patient's bottom.
- Replace bottom clothing.

- Change sheets and leave patient comfortable and safe position

Assessment of the skin

The skin can provide a great deal of information about a person's general health.
Colour – underlying disease (e.g. jaundice = liver; pallor = circulatory)
Temperature – underlying disease (fever = infection; cold = circulatory problems)
Type and texture – African = thicker cartilage and little signs of ageing; Northern European = thin skin and signs of ageing
Scars – indicating old wounds/surgical procedures
Abnormal skin conditions – rashes, lesions, pigmentations, pustules could indicate underlying pathophysiological problems
Integrity of the skin – excoriations, abrasions, risk of pressure ulcer formation

Healthy skin is defined as:
Even skin colour, smooth texture, well-hydrated and with normal sensation (no itching, burning or stinging).

Special considerations

Overwashing the skin with harsh products/too-hot water can dry the skin and lose antibacterial abilities.

Ensure creases, e.g. under breasts, groin areas, are washed and dried thoroughly.

For patients who have weakness of one side, put the affected limb into the pyjama/nightdress first.

Intravenous lines – put bag and tubing through the sleeve first followed by patient's arm.

Remember to use play techniques when attending to a child's hygiene/skin needs.

With age, elastin is lost leaving the skin loose. Skin is also more transparent and likely to break more easily.

FIGURE 4.1 Skin and hygiene

SKIN AND WOUNDS

Skin layers

The dermis, beneath the epidermis, contains tough connective tissue, hair follicles, and sweat glands. The deeper subcutaneous tissue (hypodermis) is made of fat and connective tissue.

Six types of wounds

- **Puncture:** caused by a sharp or pointed object entering skin.
- **Abrasion:** caused by scraping away the superficial layers of skin.
- **Incision:** intentional cut by sharp instrument such as a scalpel.
- **Laceration:** involves mechanical force and tearing of skin.
- **Burn:** skin erosion by heat, chemicals, radiation, or electricity.
- **Ulceration:** excavation of tissue due to sloughing away of non-viable tissue.

| Open OR Closed | Acute OR Chronic | Clean OR Contaminated |

Healing

Several stages – process the same but time fame depends on wound type:

Inflammation → Proliferation → Maturation

Factors affecting healing

- Age
- Nutrition
- Obesity
- Repeated trauma
- Skin moisture
- Chronic conditions
- Medications

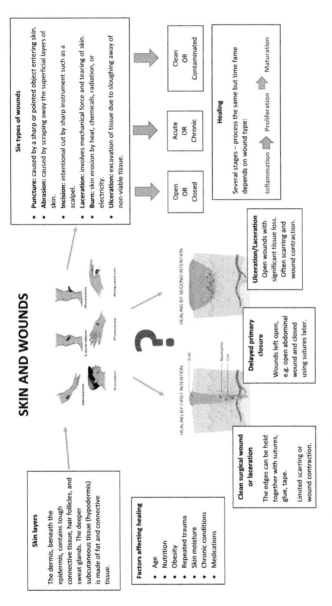

HEALING BY FIRST INTENTION

HEALING BY SECOND INTENTION

Clean surgical wound or laceration

The edges can be held together with sutures, glue, tape.

Limited scarring or wound contraction.

Delayed primary closure

Wounds left open, e.g. open abdominal wound and closed using sutures later.

Ulceration/Laceration

Open wounds with significant tissue loss. Often scarring and wound contraction.

FIGURE 4.2 Skin and wounds

WOUNDS: ASSESSMENT AND CARE

Wound assessment

Wound assessment includes:

a) Wound history
Acute, chronic, surgical

b) Type of wound
Wound classification, location and size/depth

c) Wound bed appearance and characteristics
Five main wound bed tissue types. The type of tissue present is an indication of the stage of healing or any complications present. These may include necrotic, sloughy, granulation, epithelial and hypergranulation tissue.

NB wound assessment and management can be challenging in long-term drug users, particular those who inject regularly.

Taking a wound swab

This is a frequently practiced task and needs to be done correctly to obtain the right answer to the question of types of bacteria present.

1. Prepare the required equipment (swabs, dressing packs (if needed), gloves, apron etc.).
2. Inform the patient of the need for a swab and obtain their consent.
3. Maintain hand hygiene.
4. Always clean the wound first.
5. Using the correct sterile microbiology swab, holding it with thumb and finger, rotate the swab in a zigzag direction across the wound bed.
6. Insert into the medium.
7. Label correctly with all patient's details and wound location, send to the laboratory.
8. Document in the patients nursing notes.

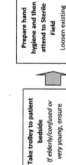

Removal of sutures: As aseptic technique using sterile equipment:

1. *Hold the knot of the suture with forceps, gently lift upwards and out to ensure it is clear of skin.*
2. *Cut one side of the suture with the stitch cutter close to the skin*
3. *Gently but firmly pull the suture out from the opposite side – DO NOT cut both sides of the knot*

IF clips:

4. *Gently place the lower two prongs under the staple or clip.*
5. *Squeeze the handles to lift the edges of the clip.*
6. *Lift one side then the other and ease out of the skin.*
7. *Clean wound and dress or as local protocol dictates.*

ASEPTIC TECHNIQUE (cleaning a wound) – Remember Wash hands BEFORE and AFTER

Prepare necessary equipment on trolley – Inform patient of the procedure and reasons.
Clean hands again. Gain consent to clean the wound.

Take trolley to patient bedside	**Prepare hand hygiene and then attend to Sterile Field**	**Observe wound**	**Draw up saline/sterile cleaning fluid**	**Do Not Disturb friable tissue**	**Place new dressing on wound**
If elderly/confused or very young, ensure verbal confirmation of understanding.	Loosen existing dressing, remove and discard.	Check colour or odour or exudate. Wash hands.	Nominate clean and dirty hands. Gently rinse wound with clean hand, non-touch technique, wipe with sterile gauze from one side to another.	Dry with sterile gauze gently – clean hand.	Secure, clear up. Wash hands.

FIGURE 4.3 Wound assessment and care

Burns (superficial)

These are pink, with blisters, and painful. Skin blanches on pressure. Should heal in 10 days with no scarring. Generally caused by scalding, electrical flash burn, radiation (sunburn).

Management aims
- Control exudate, reduce the risk of infection.
- Promote wound healing, maintain function, provide comfort.

Concern and referral is needed with patients in the following burn injuries due to potential risk with safeguarding:

- Burns in children
- Burns in adults over 60 years of age
- Burns to face, hands, feet or perineum

Fistula

This refers to an abnormal passage between two epithelial surfaces that connect one viscera (organ) to another or to the body surface, e.g. between the anal canal and skin surface.

Management aims
- Manage and encourage free drainage of the exudate.
- Reduce risk of infection.
- Promote granulation from the base of the wound.
- Remove necrosis or slough present.

RANGE OF WOUND TYPES

Who is affected?
All ages are susceptible to wounds.
Caution is needed to observe for consequences which can be life-threatening in the very young, old or other vulnerable individuals.

Open wounds

Falls, accidents with sharp objects, and car accidents are the most common causes of open wounds.

Key complications include:

Infection
See inflammation, and there may be fever

Lockjaw
Caused by an infection from the bacteria that cause tetanus. Causes muscle contractions in the jaw and neck.

Necrotizing fasciitis
This is rare but can occur: a severe soft tissue infection caused by a variety of bacteria e.g. *clostridium* and *streptococcus* This can lead to tissue loss and sepsis.

Cellulitis
A bacterial infection of the skin around a wound.

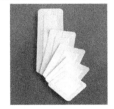

Lacerations
This refers to tearing or splitting of the skin caused by blunt trauma or an incision of the skin caused by a sharp object. The most common complication of lacerations is infection, but there may also be injuries to the underlying nerves, tissue and blood vessels. The risk of infection is increased by:
- diabetes
- visible contamination
- increasing age
- increasing time from injury to repair
- increasing depth, length and width of the laceration.

Abrasion
- This occurs when skin rubs or scrapes against a rough or hard surface. Skidding along a pavement for example.
- Usually only a small amount of bleeding, but wound may contain debris.

Puncture
- A puncture is a small hole caused by a long, pointed object, such as a nail or needle.
- These may not bleed much, but can be deep enough to damage internal organs.

Avulsion
- This is a partial or complete tearing away of skin and the tissue beneath. They occur during violent accidents for example: crushing accidents, explosions or gunshots.
- They bleed heavily and rapidly.

FIGURE 4.4 Range of wounds

WOUND CARE AND MANAGEMENT

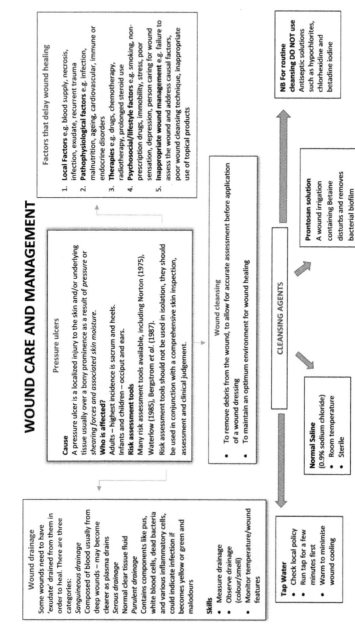

Pressure ulcers

Cause

A pressure ulcer is a localized injury to the skin and/or underlying tissue usually over a bony prominence as a result of *pressure or shearing forces and associated skin moisture*.

Who is affected?

Adults – highest incidence is sacrum and heels.
Infants and children – occiput and ears.

Risk assessment tools

Many risk assessment tools available, including Norton (1975), Waterlow (1985), Bergstrom et al. (1987).
Risk assessment tools should not be used in isolation, they should be used in conjunction with a comprehensive skin inspection, assessment and clinical judgement.

Factors that delay wound healing

1. **Local Factors** e.g. blood supply, necrosis, infection, exudate, recurrent trauma
2. **Pathophysiological factors** e.g. infection, malnutrition, ageing, cardiovascular, immune or endocrine disorders
3. **Therapies** e.g. drugs, chemotherapy, radiotherapy, prolonged steroid use
4. **Psychosocial/lifestyle factors** e.g. smoking, non-prescription drugs, immobility, stress, poor sensation, depression, person caring for wound
5. **Inappropriate wound management** e.g. failure to assess the wound and address causal factors, poor wound cleansing technique, inappropriate use of topical products

Wound drainage

Some wounds need to have 'exudate' drained from them in order to heal. There are three categories:

Sanguineous drainage
Composed of blood usually from deep wounds – may become clearer as plasma drains

Serous drainage
Normal clear tissue fluid

Purulent drainage
Contains components like pus, white blood cells, dead bacteria and various inflammatory cells, could indicate infection if becomes yellow or green and malodours

Skills

- Measure drainage
- Observe drainage (colour/smell)
- Monitor temperature/wound features

Wound cleansing

- To remove debris from the wound, to allow for accurate assessment before application of a wound dressing
- To maintain an optimum environment for wound healing

CLEANSING AGENTS

Tap Water
- Check local policy
- Run tap for a few minutes first
- Warm to minimise wound cooling

Normal Saline (0.9% sodium chloride)
- Room temperature
- Sterile

Prontosan solution
A wound irrigation containing Betaine disturbs and removes bacterial biofilm

NB For routine cleansing DO NOT use Antiseptic solutions such as hypochlorites, chlorhexidine and betadine iodine

FIGURE 4.5 Wound care and management

BANDAGING SKILLS

Bandaging

Bandages are grouped according to their material properties and functions, and fall into two broad categories:

1. Lightweight conforming stretch bandages to maintain dressing etc.
2. Substantive – cotton, elastane – main functions include support, management of sprains and strains, prevention of oedema.

Bandaging technique

- Select appropriate width of bandage and purpose – suggestions:
  - lower arm, elbow, hand and foot – 75mm
  - upper arm, knee and lower leg – 100mm
  - large leg or trunk – 150mm.
- Support the patient's limb/body part adequately before starting to apply the bandage.
- Hold the tightly rolled bandage with the 'head' of the bandage on top and wrap the 'tail' around the body part without unrolling more than a few centimetres at a time.
- Begin with a securing roll, holding the start of the bandage securely under each subsequent turn.
- Work from the narrowest part below the dressing and work upwards.
- Ensure each turn covers two-thirds of the previous turn.
- Cover totally any dressing and padding used.
- Finish with a straight turn at the end of the bandage.
- Secure the bandage with safety clip or adhesive tape. Take care if using safety pins!

Reef knots

Remember: 'right over left, then left over right'

Triangular bandage

Encourage the patient to hold the affected arm across the body in the position of greatest comfort.	Hold the triangle bandage with the base running down the centre of the body and the point to the elbow on the affected side.	Lift up the lower point and take it to meet the upper point at the side of the neck.	Tie a 'reef knot' to secure just above the collarbone to avoid any pressure to the neck.	Check the circulation in the fingers and compare the tissue colour with unaffected hand/arm.

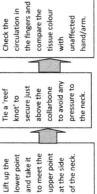

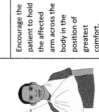

FIGURE 4.6 Bandaging skills

Activity: now test yourself

1   When taking a wound swab, which movement of the swab is recommended?:

    a   A circle of the wound bed

    b   A square around the wound edges

    c   A zigzag across the breadth of the wound

    d   No specific movement across the wound

2   Wound assessment includes all of the following EXCEPT:

    a   Wound bed

    b   Wound history

    c   Wound bed characteristics

    d   Patient factors (nutrition, etc.)

    e   Environmental features (pollution, etc.)

3   When removing sutures, it is best to cut the knot on both sides to release the suture:

    a   YES – why?

    b   NO – why?
        Why?...
        ....

4   Healing by PRIMARY INTENTION refers to what?:

    a   A clean surgical incision where the sides of the wound join with minimal loss of tissue

    b   A complex cavity wound with much loss of tissue that needs packing

    c   A complex wound involving an external object, e.g. splinters where the sides of the wound heal with no loss of tissue

    d   A simple wound with minimal dressing needed

Answers

1   c
    The z-swab technique most accurately reflects wound 'tissue' bioburden, rather than surface contamination, and provides the most clinically meaningful information. During the technique the nurse must also ensure that the swab is turning in a circular movement to totally cover the swab, while ensuring that there is minimal discomfort for the patient. This offers a representative area of the wound sample.

2   e
    All the features are correct and the environment is not a key issue unless there are some significant environmental problems, such as housing conditions (or homelessness), or if the patient is exposed to other environmental agents, such as unregulated temperature or other hazards.

3   b   NO
    The key is to remove the entire suture – by cutting either side, a portion is left within the wound and may aggravate it or lead to a local reaction or infection and be uncomfortable.

4   a
    This is a simple incised wound and the cut sides neatly adhere to each other; healing commences relatively quickly because there is no tissue loss and scarring is minimal. Complex cavity wounds have a lot of tissue loss and healing commences from the base of the wound upwards, called 'secondary intention'.

Reflection: ask yourself

1   What do I know now that I didn't know before?

2   What am I confused/unclear about?

3   What areas do I need to focus on?

4   My action plan for further learning (make objectives SMART)

Bibliography

Adams, M. and Koch, R. (2010) *Pharmacology: Connections to Nursing Practice*. Prentice Hall, NJ: Pearson.

Bergstrom, N., Braden, B.J., Laguzza, A. and Holmann, V. (1987) The Braden scale for predicting pressure sore risk. *Nurse Research* **36**(4): 205–210.

Department of Health (DoH) (2012) *Long Term Conditions: Compendium of Information*, 3rd edn. London: HMSO. Available at: www.gov.uk/government/publications/long-term-conditions-compendium-of-information-third-edition.

Guest, J.F., Vowden, K. and Vowden, P. (2017) The health economic burden that acute and chronic wounds impose on an average clinical commissioning group/health board in the UK. *Journal of Wound Care* **26**: 292–303.

Hayes, C., Jackson, D., Davidson, P.M. and Power, T. (2015) Medication errors in hospitals: a literature review of disruptions to nursing practice during medication administration. *Journal of Clinical Nursing* **24**: 3063–3076.

Health and Safety Executive (HSE) (2002) *Control of Substances Hazardous to Health (COSHH)*. London: HMSO. Available from http://www.hse.gov.uk/nanotechnology/coshh.htm (accessed 12 November 2019).

Keers, K.M., Williams, S.D., Cooke, J. and Ashcroft, D.M. (2013) Causes of medication administration errors in hospitals: A systematic review of quantitative and qualitative evidence. *Drug Safety* **36**: 1045–1067.

Loveday, H.P., Wilson, J.A., Pratt, R.J. *et al.* (2014) epic3: National evidence-based guidelines for preventing healthcare-associated infections in NHS hospitals in England. *Journal of Hospital Infection* **86**(Suppl 1): S1–S70.

Medicines Act (1968) London: HMSO. Available at: www.legislation.gov.uk/ukpga/1968/67 (accessed 11 November 2019).

Medicines and Healthcare Regulatory Authority (MHRA) (2017) *Rules and Guidance for Pharmaceutical Manufacturers and Distributors*. London: Pharmaceutical Press.

Misuse of Drugs Regulations (2001) London: HMSO. Available at: www.legislation.gov.uk/uksi/2001/3998/contents/made (accessed 11 November 2019).

National Health Service (NHS) (2016) *The Routine Immunisation Schedule.* London: HMSO.

National Institute for Clinical and Healthcare Excellence (NICE) (2012) *Older People: Independence and mental wellbeing.* NICE guideline [NG32]. Available at: www.nice.org.uk/guidance/ng32.

National Institute for Health and Care Excellence (NICE) (2014) *Infection Prevention and Control. Quality standard* [QS61]. London: NICE. Available at: www.nice.org.uk/guidance/QS61/chapter/Introduction.

National Institute for Health and Care Excellence (NICE) (2015) *Medicines Optimisation: The safe and effective use of medicines to enable the best possible outcomes.* NICE guidelines. Available at: nice.org.uk/guidance/ng5.

Norton, D., McLaren, R. and Exton-Smith, A.N. (1975) *An Investigation of Geriatric Nursing Problems in Hospital.* Edinburgh: Churchill Livingstone.

Nursing and Midwifery Council (NMC) (2007) *Standards for Medicines Management.* London. NMC.

Nursing and Midwifery Council (NMC) (2018a) *Future Nurse Proficiencies.* London: NMC. Available at: www.nmc.org.uk/standards/standards-for-nurses/standards-of-proficiency-for-registered-nurses (accessed 1 May 2019).

Nursing and Midwifery Council (NMC) (2018b) *The Code: Professional Standards of Practice and Behaviou*r. London: NMC.

O'Driscoll, B.R., Howard, L.S., Earis, J. and Mak, V., on behalf of the British Thoracic Society Emergency Oxygen Guideline Development Group (BTS) (2017) British Thoracic Society Guidelines for Oxygen in Adults in Healthcare and Emergency Settings (online). Available at: http://bmjopenrespres.bmj.com (accessed 11 November 2019).

Public Health England (PHE) (2016) Point Prevalence Survey of Healthcare Associated Infections, Antimicrobial Use and Antimicrobial Stewardship in England: Protocol gateway. London: Public Health England.

Public Health England (PHE) (2018) Mandatory *Healthcare Associated Infection Surveillance: Data Quality Statement.* London: Public Health England. Available at: https://assets.publishing.service.gov.uk/government/uploads/system/uploads/attachment_data/file/713604/Mandatory_Healthcare_Associated_Infection_Surveillance_Data_Quality_Statement.pdf.

Resuscitation Council (UK) (2015) Resuscitation guidelines (online). Available at: www.resus.org.uk/resuscitation-guidelines (accessed 19 May 2019).

Royal College of Nursing (RCN) (2018) *Tools of the Trade.* London: RCN.

Royal Pharmaceutical Society (RPS) (2016) *A Competency Framework for all Prescribers*. London: Royal Pharmaceutical Society.

Royal Pharmaceutical Society (RPS) (2019) *Professional Guidance on the Administration of Medicines in Healthcare Settings*. London. Royal Pharmaceutical Society. Available at: www.rpharms.com/Portals/0/RPS%20document%20library/Open%20access/Professional%20standards/SSHM%20and%20Admin/Admin%20of%20Meds%20prof%20guidance.pdf?ver=2019-01-23-145026-567

Waterlow, J. (1985) Pressure sores: A risk assessment card. *Nursing Times* 81(48):49–95.

Willcock, J. and Jewkes F. (2000) Making sense of fluid balance in children. *Peadiatric Nursing* **12**(7):37–42.

World Health Organization (WHO) (2009) *WHO Guidelines on Hand Hygiene in Health Care*. Geneva: WHO. Available at: https://apps.who.int/iris/bitstream/handle/10665/44102/9789241597906_eng.pdf;jsessionid=09BB349AD9998F3342A3ED29D72116D9?sequence=1 (accessed 12 November 2019).

Index

Page numbers in *italics* denote figures.

INDEX

For Product Safety Concerns and Information please contact our EU
representative GPSR@taylorandfrancis.com Taylor & Francis Verlag GmbH,
Kaufingerstraße 24, 80331 München, Germany

Printed and bound by CPI Group (UK) Ltd, Croydon, CR0 4YY
01/05/2025
01858520-0001